COMPLETE GUIDE TO INFLAMMATORY BOWEL DISEASE

Comprehensive Handbook For Understanding, Managing, Thriving, Treatment Strategies, Diet Plans, And Lifestyle Tips Included

DEHART HAIRSTON

DISCLAIMER

This book's content is only intended for general informative purposes. At the time of writing, the author has taken every precaution to guarantee that the material is correct and current. Nevertheless, the author disclaims all explicit and implicit representations and guarantees about the availability, appropriateness, correctness, completeness, and usefulness of the material on these pages.

Since the author is not a licensed medical practitioner, the material in this book shouldn't be interpreted as medical advice. Before making any modifications to their diet, exercise regimen, or medical treatment, readers are urged to speak with a licensed healthcare provider.

Moreover, the author has no connection to any of the businesses, organizations, or people that are discussed in this book. Any mentions of goods, services, businesses, or people are purely informative and do not indicate endorsement or suggestion.

This book's content is entirely dependent on the author's expertise, study, and comprehension of the topic. Despite having taken reasonable care to offer correct information, the author disclaims all liability for any mistakes or omissions in the material as well as for any losses, harm, or damages resulting from using the information.

It is recommended that readers use their own judgment and discretion when applying the knowledge in this book to their own situations. The use or implementation of any material in this book may result in unfavorable repercussions, directly or indirectly, for which the author assumes no liability.

By reading this book, you agree to release and hold the author harmless from any claims, losses, liabilities, costs, or expenditures resulting from or related to the use of the information you get from it.

ABOUT THE BOOK

"Inflammatory Bowel Disease" is more than simply a book; it's a thorough manual that enables those struggling with this difficult illness to make sense of their path. This book's well-written information makes it an invaluable resource for healthcare providers, patients, and caregivers alike.

The first step in treating Inflammatory Bowel Disease (IBD) properly is understanding it, and Chapter 1 lays the groundwork by explaining the nuances of this ailment. The many forms of IBD are explained, along with its origins and symptoms, giving readers essential knowledge about their illness.

Initiating appropriate care requires a diagnosis, which is why Chapter 2 explores the range of diagnostic techniques that are accessible. From medical history to endoscopic treatments, readers will have the information necessary to interact more productively with their healthcare professionals.

Chapter 3 provides a thorough summary of the many treatment options available, ranging from medicine to surgical treatments. As this chapter explains, lifestyle adjustments can have a significant impact.

The difficulties of having IBD are unique, and Chapter 4 discusses coping techniques, support systems, and methods for preserving a good standard of living.

Nutrition and diet play a major role in controlling IBD, and Chapter 5 gives readers the tools they need to make educated decisions by offering helpful advice on meal planning and food selection.

Chapter 6 demystifies the complex process of medication management, covering everything from comprehending drugs to tracking the efficacy of therapy.

IBD is often accompanied by comorbidities and related disorders; Chapter 7 provides information on possible complications, extraintestinal symptoms, and preventative actions.

Chapter 8 discusses pharmaceutical safety, illness management throughout pregnancy, and fertility issues for people thinking about becoming pregnant or starting a family.

The management of IBD advances due to research and inventions; Chapter 9 examines these developments, possible treatments, and patient involvement in clinical trials.

As Chapter 10 emphasizes, raising awareness and promoting advocacy is crucial for building support and accelerating change.

CHAPTER 1

Understanding Inflammatory Bowel Disease

What Is Inflammatory Bowel Disease?

The term "inflammatory bowel disease" (IBD) refers to a collection of gastrointestinal tract-related chronic inflammatory diseases. Since IBD and IBS (Irritable Bowel Syndrome) are two separate disorders, it's important to distinguish between the two. Ulcerative colitis and Crohn's disease are the two primary forms of IBD. The gastrointestinal (GI) tract is inflamed in these disorders, which may lead to a variety of symptoms and problems.

Types Of Inflammatory Bowel Disease: Crohn's Disease And Ulcerative Colitis

Inflammatory bowel disease

Any portion of the digestive system, from the mouth to the anus, may be affected by Crohn's disease, but the ileum (the end of the small intestine) and the colon (the beginning of the large intestine) are where it most often manifests. Deep intestinal wall penetration by the inflammation associated with Crohn's disease may result in issues such as fistulas, irregular connections between various portions of the intestine, and strictures, or constriction of the gut.

Colitis Ulcerative:

The colon and rectum are most affected by ulcerative colitis. The inflammation associated with Ulcerative Colitis is restricted to the inner lining of the colon and rectum, in contrast to Crohn's Disease, which may affect any region of the digestive system. Usually beginning in the rectum, this inflammation steadily moves up the colon. It may result in the development of ulcers, or sores, in the colon's lining, which can produce symptoms including bloody diarrhea, discomfort in the abdomen, and a sudden need to go to the bathroom.

Causes And Risk Factors

Although the precise origin of inflammatory bowel disease is unknown, immune system, environmental, and genetic variables are thought to be involved. IBD tends to run in families, therefore genetics play a big part. Environmental elements like stress, food, smoking, and infections may also play a role in the development of IBD. Furthermore, immune system anomalies—in which the immune system of the body unintentionally targets the digestive tract—are believed to be a major contributor to the development of inflammation.

The following risk factors raise the possibility of getting IBD:

• Family history: Your risk is increased if you have a close family who has IBD.

• Age: While IBD may strike at any age, it usually starts in adolescence or the early stages of adulthood.

• Ethnicity: Ashkenazi Jews, for example, are more likely to acquire IBD than other ethnic groups.

• Smoking: While smoking tends to protect against ulcerative colitis, it is a substantial risk factor for Crohn's disease.

• Environmental factors: Residing in developed nations or metropolitan regions may raise your chance of getting IBD.

Signs And Symptoms

Depending on the kind of IBD and the degree of inflammation, different IBD signs and symptoms may appear. Typical signs and symptoms include:

• Prolonged diarrhea

• Cramps and discomfort in the abdomen

• Bleeding in the rectal area

• The need for a quick bowel movement

• Loss of weight

• Tiredness

• High temperature

• Appetite loss

It is important to understand that symptoms may change over time, alternating between times of active illness (flare-ups) and periods of remission (few or no symptoms). To control symptoms and stop flare-ups, a mix of medication, lifestyle modifications, and sometimes surgery is used. For people with inflammatory bowel disease to have better results and a higher quality of life, early diagnosis and treatment are essential.

CHAPTER 2

Diagnosing Inflammatory Bowel Disease

Medical History And Physical Examination

A thorough medical history and physical examination are often the first steps in the diagnosis of inflammatory bowel disease (IBD). Your doctor will review your past medical history and pay particular attention to any symptoms you have had, such as weariness, diarrhea, stomach discomfort, and weight loss. They will also ask about any relevant medical history you may have, such as autoimmune illnesses, digestive disorders, or other ailments.

Your doctor will probably palpate your belly to feel for any soreness, listen to your bowel movements, and look for any irregularities or indications of inflammation during the physical examination.

They could also evaluate your dietary state and general health.

Important hints are provided by this first evaluation to direct further diagnostic procedures. It's important to keep in mind, too, that accurate IBD diagnosis often requires a mix of several tests and treatments.

Laboratory Tests And Imaging Studies

To diagnose IBD, laboratory testing is essential. Certain biomarkers linked to inflammation, such as erythrocyte sedimentation rate (ESR) and C-reactive protein (CRP), may be found in blood testing. Increased concentrations of these indicators could point to the body's ongoing inflammation.

Blood tests may also evaluate your general health, including iron, vitamin B12, and folate deficits—

nutrient deficiencies that are frequent in people with IBD.

Another crucial instrument in the diagnosis procedure is imaging studies. A thorough picture of the gastrointestinal system may be obtained using methods including X-rays, CT scans, and magnetic resonance imaging (MRI), which can be used to spot anomalies such as fistulas, strictures, and inflammation.

In some instances, your medical professional could suggest specialized imaging tests to get a better image of certain digestive system regions, including a barium swallow or barium enema.

Laboratory tests and imaging investigations, when paired with the data gleaned from your physical examination and medical history, can provide a thorough assessment of your health that will influence future testing and treatment decisions.

Endoscopic Procedures

Endoscopic techniques play a crucial role in the diagnosis and assessment of inflammatory bowel disease (IBD). The most often used endoscopic techniques for identifying inflammatory bowel disease (IBD) are colonoscopy and esophagogastroduodenoscopy (EGD).

A flexible, illuminated tube called a colonoscope—which has a camera—is moved into the colon and placed into the rectum during a colonoscopy. This enables the medical professional to see the colon's lining and see any inflammation, ulcers, or other irregularities that are indicative of IBD.

In a similar vein, an endoscope is inserted via the mouth into the duodenum, stomach, and esophagus during an endoscopy. This treatment aids in evaluating the upper gastrointestinal tract for anomalies that could point to IBD, such as ulcers or symptoms of inflammation.

In the process of diagnosing and classifying IBD, tissue samples (biopsies) may be taken for further examination. via microscopic examination of the tissue, pathologists may discover particular traits associated with Crohn's disease or ulcerative colitis via biopsies.

Not only are endoscopic procedures essential for the diagnosis of inflammatory bowel disease (IBD), but they also monitor the illness's activity throughout time, support treatment choices, and evaluate the effectiveness of therapy.

Biopsy And Histological Examination

Histological analysis and biopsy are essential steps in the IBD diagnosis process. Samples of tissue taken during endoscopic procedures can distinguish between ulcerative colitis and Crohn's disease and provide important insights into the underlying pathophysiology.

To detect hallmark signs of IBD, such as inflammation, crypt distortion, epithelial damage, and architectural alterations in the intestinal mucosa, tissue samples are examined under a microscope in a process known as histological examination.

For instance, transmural inflammation and granuloma development are common histological findings in Crohn's disease, although diffuse inflammation restricted to the mucosal layer is usual in ulcerative colitis.

These histological differences help to inform prognosis and treatment choices in addition to helping to confirm the diagnosis. Furthermore, histological examination may reveal other gastrointestinal disorders or consequences that resemble IBD, guaranteeing precise diagnosis and suitable treatment.

In conclusion, biopsy and histological examination are crucial add-ons to endoscopic procedures in the diagnosis of inflammatory bowel disease (IBD), offering vital data that influences patient treatment and enhances results.

CHAPTER 3

Treatment Options

Medications For Managing Symptoms

Medication is an essential part of treating the symptoms of inflammatory bowel disease (IBD). Several drug options address various facets of the ailment.

1. Aminosalicylates: These drugs function to lessen intestinal lining irritation. When it comes to mild to moderate instances of IBD, especially ulcerative colitis, they are often the first to intervene. Aminosalicylates are available as oral tablets, capsules, and enemas, among other forms.

2. Corticosteroids: During flare-ups, corticosteroids, which are strong anti-inflammatory medications, are usually used for the temporary alleviation of moderate to severe symptoms.

Though they can decrease inflammation immediately, their possible adverse effects, including mood fluctuations, weight gain, and loss of bone density, make them unsuitable for long-term usage.

3. Immunomodulators: These drugs function by reducing the aberrant immune response that causes IBD-related inflammation in the body. To sustain remission and lessen the need for corticosteroids, they are often used in conjunction with other drugs. It might take a few weeks or months for immunomodulators to start working.

4. Biologic Therapies: Biologic medications target certain immune system proteins that contribute to the inflammatory process of inflammatory bowel disease (IBD). Usually, they are reserved for moderate-to-severe IBD patients when previous therapies have not worked satisfactorily. In many cases, biologics may successfully induce and sustain remission when given by injection or infusion.

5. **Antibiotics:** Infections may be treated with antibiotics, and they can also be used to help control Crohn's disease consequences such as fistulas and abscesses. Although they are not usually the first line of therapy for IBD, they could be in certain circumstances.

It's important to collaborate closely with your healthcare practitioner to identify the best drug schedule for your particular illness and to keep an eye out for any possible problems or side effects.

Diet And Nutrition Strategies

Although there isn't one diet that works for everyone with IBD, there are dietary approaches that may help control symptoms and enhance general health.

1. Low-residue Diet: This kind of diet restricts high-fiber foods such as nuts, seeds, and fresh fruits and vegetables. This might lessen pain and decrease bowel motions during flare-ups.

2. Elimination Diet: By figuring out which foods to avoid, some people with IBD can reduce their symptoms. Keeping a diet journal and progressively reintroducing foods may be necessary to identify which ones are troublesome.

3. Nutritional Supplements: To guarantee sufficient consumption of vital vitamins and minerals in situations where malnutrition or nutrient shortages are evident, nutritional supplements may be advised. This may promote general well-being and recovery.

4. Probiotics: Probiotics are good bacteria that may aid in reestablishing the gut microbiome's equilibrium.

Some studies indicate that certain probiotic strains may help lower inflammation and improve symptoms in people with IBD, but further study is required to confirm this.

5. Fluid Intake: Everyone needs to stay hydrated, but it's particularly critical for those with IBD who may get dehydrated or have diarrhea. Throughout the day, drinking plenty of water may help avoid problems and enhance general health.

Working with a licensed dietitian or nutritionist who specializes in IBD is crucial if you want to create a customized eating plan that suits your tastes and requirements.

Surgical Interventions

Surgical intervention could be required in some situations to control problems or enhance the quality of life for IBD patients.

1. **Strictureplasty:** This surgical technique is used to expand intestinal segments that have been restricted due to scar tissue (strictures). It may enhance digestive function and assist reduce symptoms like bowel blockage.

2. **Bowel Resection:** A bowel resection is a procedure used to remove a section of the intestine that has been seriously damaged or diseased. By doing so, symptoms may be lessened and problems like fistulas or abscesses may be avoided.

3. **Colectomy:** A colectomy is a surgical procedure in which the colon is removed whole or in part. If a patient develops issues like toxic megacolon or colon cancer, or if their severe ulcerative colitis does not improve with medication, it could be advised.

4. **Ostomy Surgery:** An ostomy may be produced in some situations, especially when a significant piece

of the colon or rectum is removed. This entails making a surgical incision (stoma) in the belly so that waste may be expelled and placed into an external pouch.

5. J-Pouch Surgery: To build a new reservoir for the body to store feces, a J-pouch surgery may be done on patients who have had a colectomy. This allows for more regular bowel movement by forming the end of the small intestine into a pouch that is attached to the rectum or anus.

Usually, surgical procedures are reserved for situations in which medicinal treatment has failed or in which difficulties have developed. To make an educated choice, you must talk to your healthcare professional about the advantages and disadvantages of surgery.

Lifestyle Modifications

Apart from pharmaceutical and surgical interventions, lifestyle changes may significantly aid in the management of inflammatory bowel disease and enhance the general standard of living.

1. Effective stress management is essential because stress may aggravate the symptoms of inflammatory bowel disease (IBD). This might include asking friends, family, or a therapist for help in addition to practicing relaxation methods like yoga, meditation, or deep breathing.

2. Frequent Exercise: Research has shown that exercise may help people with IBD feel better emotionally, decrease inflammation, and enhance their general well-being. To get the most advantages, try to combine cardiovascular, strength, and flexibility activities.

3. Quitting Smoking: It is well established that smoking increases the chance of getting Crohn's disease. It may also exacerbate symptoms and reduce the efficacy of certain treatments. One of the most crucial things you can do to control your illness and enhance your health is to stop smoking.

4. Sufficient Sleep: Insufficient sleep may exacerbate IBD symptoms and lead to inflammation. By adopting healthy sleep hygiene practices, such as adhering to a regular sleep schedule, establishing a calming bedtime ritual, and optimizing your sleeping environment, you may aim for seven to nine hours of excellent sleep every night.

5. Avoiding Trigger Factors: Recognize and stay away from things that make your symptoms flare up, such as certain meals, drugs, or surroundings. You may take proactive measures to reduce the effect of triggers on your health by tracking trends and identifying them with the use of a symptom diary.

Together with the right medical and surgical care, you may improve your quality of life and effectively manage your IBD by implementing these lifestyle changes into your daily routine. Always get advice from your healthcare practitioner before making any big adjustments to your treatment regimen or way of life.

CHAPTER 4

Living With Inflammatory Bowel Disease

Coping With Flares And Managing Stress

Handling flare-ups and stress management are two of the most difficult elements of having Inflammatory Bowel Disease (IBD). Periods of increased symptoms including exhaustion, diarrhea, and stomach discomfort are known as flares, and they may seriously interfere with day-to-day activities. Nonetheless, there are methods to lessen their effects and enhance general well-being.

Above all, it's critical to identify the warning indicators of an approaching flare. This entails keeping an eye out for any signs that can point to the presence of the illness, such as altered bowel habits, increased tiredness, and abdominal discomfort.

IBD patients may often reduce the severity of a flare by being watchful and proactive in their interventions.

Controlling stress is essential for controlling IBD flare-ups. It has been shown that stress makes many IBD sufferers' symptoms worse and may set off flare-ups. Thus, learning practical stress-reduction methods is essential. This might include indulging in relaxing and joyful hobbies and activities, as well as techniques like yoga, deep breathing exercises, and mindfulness meditation. Joining support groups or obtaining assistance from mental health specialists may also provide helpful coping strategies and techniques for stress management.

During a flare-up, dietary changes may also help reduce symptoms. Although there isn't a single diet that works for everyone with IBD, some people find relief by cutting out certain trigger foods, including dairy, spicy foods, or high-fiber meals, for a short while. A certified dietician with expertise in IBD consultations may provide individualized advice and meal plans catered to specific requirements.

Support Networks And Resources

Although having IBD might sometimes make you feel alone, it's important to know that you are not. Creating a network of friends, family, medical professionals, and other IBD sufferers may be a great way to get support and understanding. Both in-person and virtual support groups provide people the chance to interact with others who have gone through similar things, give and receive emotional support, and trade advice.

For those with IBD, there are a plethora of options accessible in addition to peer support. To empower people and their families, organizations like the Crohn's & Colitis Foundation provide educational materials, webinars, and advocacy tools. These groups often organize walks or fundraising campaigns, offering chances for community involvement and IBD awareness-raising.

Healthcare professionals are a vital component of your support system as well. Establishing a trustworthy rapport with your gastroenterologist, nurse practitioner, or other healthcare team members is crucial for efficiently treating your illness. Never be afraid to express concerns, ask questions, or seek clarity on your treatment plan.

Maintaining Quality Of Life

Even if having IBD comes with obstacles, it's important to give priority to pursuits and routines that enhance general health and quality of life.

This entails leading a well-balanced lifestyle that includes consistent exercise, enough sleep, and stress reduction practices.

The difficulties of having a chronic disease may be lessened by engaging in happy and fulfilling activities. Setting aside time for pursuits that feed the soul—such as helping in the community, engaging in hobbies and interests, or spending time with loved ones—is crucial to preserving optimism and fortitude in the face of hardship.

Mental and emotional well-being may also be enhanced by self-care techniques including frequent self-reflection, establishing boundaries, and cultivating appreciation. It's important to pay attention to your body's needs and make self-care activities a priority to replenish your energy and foster harmony and balance in your life.

Communicating With Healthcare Providers

To properly manage IBD, good contact with medical professionals is crucial. Developing a cooperative connection with your nurse practitioner, gastroenterologist, and other healthcare team members guarantees that you will have the assistance and direction you need to effectively manage your problem.

Talk to your healthcare professional about your concerns, treatment choices, and symptoms as soon as possible. Maintain a symptom diary to document any changes in your health as well as any patterns or triggers you become aware of. This might assist your healthcare practitioner in customizing your treatment plan to suit your choices and requirements.

Never be afraid to clarify anything you don't understand about your diagnosis, available treatments, or any other element of your care. At every step of the process, your healthcare practitioner is there to assist and advise you. Together, you may create a thorough treatment plan that targets your requirements and objectives for successfully controlling IBD.

CHAPTER 5

Diet And Nutrition

Understanding The Role Of Diet In Inflammatory Bowel Disease

When it comes to treating Inflammatory Bowel Disease (IBD), which encompasses ulcerative colitis and Crohn's disease, diet is essential. Although nutrition cannot treat IBD on its own, it may have a big influence on managing symptoms and general well-being. Creating a diet plan that is optimal for symptom management and healing requires an understanding of how certain foods impact the digestive system.

IBD is characterized by inflammation and damage to the gastrointestinal tract as a result of the immune system attacking it in error. While certain meals may help lessen symptoms and encourage recovery, others may either cause or exacerbate inflammation. IBD may also affect the body's capacity to absorb nutrients, thus it's critical to concentrate on eating a diet high in nutrients to avoid shortages.

Recommended Foods And Nutrients

Including foods high in nutrients in your diet may help control the symptoms of IBD and promote general health. Several essential nutrients to consider are:

1. **Fiber:** Although meals rich in fiber are typically better for digestion, they may make IBD flare-up symptoms worse. Soluble fibers are kinder on the digestive tract and may be found in fruits, vegetables, and cereals.

2. **Protein:** Protein is necessary for immunological response and tissue repair. Lean protein options that are less prone to irritate your skin include fish, poultry, eggs, and tofu.

3. Omega-3 Fatty Acids: The body's natural inflammatory response may be lessened by these anti-inflammatory lipids. Include foods like walnuts, chia seeds, flaxseeds, and fatty fish (salmon, mackerel) in your diet.

4. Calcium and vitamin D deficiency may be more likely in those using IBD medicines and consuming fewer dairy products. To promote bone health, include leafy greens, fortified meals, and supplements as required.

5. Fluids: Drinking enough water is crucial for controlling IBD symptoms, particularly diarrhea. Water is the best beverage to have during the day; avoid coffee and alcohol as they might exacerbate symptoms.

Foods To Avoid Or Limit

Some foods may exacerbate IBD symptoms by causing inflammation. Although each person's triggers are unique, some typical offenders include:

1. **High-Fat Foods:** Foods that are greasy or fried might be hard to digest, which can lead to upset stomach and diarrhea. Reduce your consumption of processed foods, creamy sauces, and fatty meats.

2. **Dairy Products:** People with IBD often have lactose intolerance, and dairy products may aggravate symptoms including gas, diarrhea, and bloating. Choose low-lactose dairy products in moderation or think about lactose-free substitutes.

3. **rich-Fiber Foods:** Nuts, whole grains, and raw fruits and vegetables are examples of foods rich in fiber that might exacerbate symptoms during flare-ups.

Scoop off the seeds and rough skins, cook or peel fruits and vegetables, and choose refined grains.

4. Spicy meals: For some IBD sufferers, spicy meals may aggravate their digestive system and cause inflammation. If spicy foods, sauces, and spices aggravate symptoms, cut down or stay away from them.

5. Alcohol and caffeine: These two substances have the potential to aggravate GI symptoms such as diarrhea by stimulating the digestive tract. Restrict alcohol and caffeine consumption, particularly while experiencing flare-ups.

Meal Planning Tips

Making a well-balanced food plan may boost general health and aid in the management of IBD symptoms.

Here are some pointers to think about:

1.   Maintain   a   Food   Diary: Monitor your consumption of food and symptoms to find any trends or possible causes. This will enable you to choose the items you should eat and avoid with knowledge.

2. Eat Small, Often: Choose to eat smaller, more frequent meals throughout the day as opposed to three big ones. By doing so, symptoms like bloating and pain may be reduced and the digestive system's risk of overloading is reduced.

3. Emphasis on Variety: To make sure you're receiving enough vitamins and minerals, include a variety of nutrient-rich foods in your diet. To keep meals interesting, try experimenting with tastes, textures, and cooking techniques.

4. Eat mindfully by taking your time, chewing your meal well, and enjoying every taste. To facilitate digestion and help you identify when you're full, eating slowly and carefully may assist you avoid overindulging.

5. **Speak with a Registered Dietitian:** An experienced registered dietitian with knowledge of IBD can provide you with individualized nutritional guidance and assist in creating a meal plan that suits your unique requirements and tastes.

People may enhance their overall quality of life and more effectively manage their IBD symptoms by learning how nutrition plays a key part in controlling the disease, making educated food choices, and putting practical meal-planning skills into practice.

CHAPTER 6

Medication Management

Overview Of Medications Used In Inflammatory Bowel Disease

Medication is an essential part of the management of inflammatory bowel disease (IBD) since it helps to keep symptoms under control and avoid flare-ups. Knowing the many kinds of drugs that are available will enable you and your healthcare professional to decide on your treatment strategy with knowledge.

1. Aminosalicylates: These drugs, which include mesalamine, sulfasalazine, and olsalazine, function by lessening intestinal lining irritation. They are often used to treat IBD, especially ulcerative colitis, in mild to moderate instances. Aminosalicylates come in several forms, such as enemas, suppositories, and oral tablets.

2.   **Corticosteroids:** Strong anti-inflammatory medications that may rapidly reduce symptoms during flare-ups include corticosteroids such as budesonide and prednisone. However, since they have the potential to cause major adverse effects, such as weight gain, osteoporosis, and increased infection risk, with continued usage, they are usually used for short-term relief.

3.   **Immunomodulators:** Medications such as methotrexate, azathioprine, and 6-mercaptopurine suppresses the aberrant immune response that causes inflammation in inflammatory bowel disease (IBD). When previous therapies have failed or in situations of moderate to severe IBD, these drugs are often utilized. But it might take a few weeks or months for them to have full effect.

4.   **Biologic Therapies:** Biologic medications target certain molecules involved in the inflammatory process. Examples of these

medications include ustekinumab, vedolizumab, adalimumab, and infliximab. Usually, they are reserved for moderate-to-severe IBD patients when previous therapies haven't worked successfully. For many individuals, biologics may result in long-term remission when given via injection or infusion.

5. Antibiotics: To treat infections or IBD-related problems like fistulas or abscesses, doctors may sometimes prescribe antibiotics like metronidazole and ciprofloxacin. In certain circumstances, they may also aid in reducing inflammation.

6. Painkillers and Antidiarrheal Drugs: While over-the-counter painkillers like acetaminophen and antidiarrheal drugs like loperamide may aid in the management of symptoms like diarrhea and stomach discomfort, they cannot be used as a replacement for addressing the underlying inflammation associated with inflammatory bowel disease.

 To help decrease inflammation and encourage intestinal repair, some people with IBD may benefit from nutritional therapy in addition to conventional medicine. This kind of therapy includes following a certain diet or taking nutritional supplements.

Knowing the various IBD drugs and how they function will help you and your doctor decide on the best course of action depending on your symptoms, the severity of your illness, and your personal preferences.

Understanding Side Effects And Risks

Although inflammatory bowel disease (IBD) drugs may be very helpful in managing symptoms and averting flare-ups, there may be dangers and adverse effects that should be carefully evaluated.

1. **Common adverse Effects:** Depending on the individual medicine, several drugs used to treat IBD

may have common adverse effects. For instance, corticosteroids might result in weight gain, mood fluctuations, and sleeplessness, but aminosalicylates can induce headaches, nausea, and rash. Knowing these possible side effects may help you and your healthcare practitioner prepare for and successfully manage them.

2. Significant Risks: Certain IBD drugs come with more significant side effects that need to be closely monitored in addition to the usual adverse effects. For example, prolonged usage of corticosteroids may raise the risk of diabetes, high blood pressure, and osteoporosis. Biologic treatments and immunomodulators may weaken the immune system, increasing a person's susceptibility to infections.

3. Monitoring and Surveillance: To identify any possible side effects or problems early on, regular monitoring and surveillance are crucial while taking drugs for IBD. To evaluate your general health and the efficacy of the drug, this may include imaging scans, blood tests, and other diagnostic procedures.

4. Patient Education: People with inflammatory bowel disease (IBD) must understand the risks and possible adverse effects of the drugs they take. This involves being aware of the early warning indicators of major issues and knowing when to see a doctor. Addressing any worries or inquiries you may have about your treatment plan requires an open conversation between you and your healthcare practitioner.

5. Risk-Benefit Assessment: Medical professionals carefully consider the possible risks and advantages of therapy for each patient before recommending medicine for IBD. To maximize the positive benefits of therapy while reducing negative ones, variables like the severity of the condition, prior treatment history, and general health are taken into account.

You may collaborate with your healthcare team to make educated choices about your treatment plan and minimize any possible consequences by being aware of the risks and probable side effects of IBD drugs.

Adherence Strategies

For inflammatory bowel disease (IBD) to be adequately managed and for symptoms to be under long-term control and remission, medication regimen adherence is crucial. However, adherence may be difficult to maintain for a variety of reasons, such as complicated dose regimens, side effects from medications, and lifestyle issues. Adherence-boosting tactics have the potential to greatly improve treatment results and IBD patients' quality of life.

1. Information and Counseling: It is essential to provide patients with thorough information and

counseling about their IBD and the significance of medication adherence. This entails outlining each drug's intended use, possible adverse effects, and role in managing the illness. Resolving any issues or misunderstandings may boost treatment commitment and enthusiasm.

2. Simplify Regimens: Patients may find it easier to follow their treatment plan if their pharmaceutical regimens are made simpler by employing combination treatments, lowering the number of tablets, or decreasing the frequency of doses. This might include moving to once-daily dosing, switching to extended-release versions, or tracking dosages using medication organizers.

3. Frequent Follow-up and Monitoring: Making follow-up meetings with medical professionals enables continuous evaluation of the effectiveness and tolerance of medications. Any challenges or obstacles to adherence may be found and quickly resolved during these visits. In addition, changes to the treatment plan may be made as necessary in response to the patient's condition and level of activity.

4. Employ Reminder Systems: Patients may maintain adherence to their prescription regimen by using reminder systems, such as pill organizers, smartphone applications, or alarms. Adherence may be increased by encouraging patients to include taking their medications into regular schedules, such as connecting them to mealtimes or bedtimes.

5. Address Obstacles and Difficulties: It's critical to recognize and take steps to overcome certain obstacles and difficulties that may arise from adherence, such as budgetary limitations, transportation problems, or psychological troubles. Healthcare professionals and patients may collaborate to create workable solutions and support networks to get over these challenges.

6. Involve Family and Support Networks: Patients with IBD may benefit from extra responsibility and encouragement when family members, caregivers, or support networks are included in the adherence process. A supportive atmosphere may be created by informing close ones about the significance of medication adherence and asking for their help with medication management.

Healthcare practitioners may enhance treatment results for patients with inflammatory bowel disease and maximize drug adherence by customizing adherence methods and attending to the unique requirements of each patient.

Monitoring And Adjusting Treatment

Keeping an eye on disease activity and modifying treatment plans are essential to properly treating inflammatory bowel disease (IBD). Frequent evaluation enables medical professionals to assess therapy response, spot disease progression or consequences, and make the required adjustments to improve patient outcomes.

1. Clinical Evaluation: Using the patient's medical history, physical examination, and symptom questionnaires, clinical evaluation of IBD entails assessing symptoms, disease activity, and general well-being. Standardized scoring systems, such as the Simple Clinical Colitis Activity Index (SCCAI) or the Crohn's Disease Activity Index (CDAI), may be used by healthcare professionals to measure the severity of a patient's condition and track changes over time.

2. Laboratory Testing: A variety of laboratory tests may provide important information regarding inflammation levels, nutritional health, and possible consequences of inflammatory bowel disease (IBD).

These procedures include blood tests, stool studies, and inflammatory markers including fecal calprotectin and C-reactive protein (CRP). Frequent monitoring of these markers aids in evaluating therapy response and directing therapeutic choices.

3. Imaging Studies: To see the intestinal mucosa, diagnose illness complications (like strictures or fistulas), and track the course of the disease or its response to therapy, imaging modalities including endoscopy, colonoscopy, and imaging scans (like MRI, CT scan) are crucial. These examinations may be carried out regularly or when required by clinical criteria.

4. Evaluation of Treatment Objectives: For IBD, treatment objectives usually include controlling symptoms, bringing the condition into and staying in remission, avoiding complications, and enhancing quality of life.

Healthcare professionals work with patients to create personalized treatment plans and monitor their progress regularly.

5. Medication Optimization: To improve illness management, healthcare professionals may need to change the doses of medications, use complementary therapies, or switch to other therapies based on continuous monitoring and assessment. This might include switching to biologic medications for refractory illness, increasing immunosuppressive treatment, or reducing corticosteroid dosage.

6. Multidisciplinary Approach: To fully address the wide range of demands of individuals with IBD, managing the condition often necessitates a multidisciplinary

approach including gastroenterologists, dietitians, psychologists, and other experts. Working together, healthcare professionals can better deliver individualized treatment plans, holistic care, and joint decision-making.

Healthcare practitioners may improve the management of inflammatory bowel disease and maximize outcomes by proactively adjusting treatment regimens based on routine monitoring of disease activity, treatment response, and possible consequences. Patients get individualized care and get the greatest results for their illnesses thanks to this iterative process of monitoring and therapy adjustment.

CHAPTER 7

Complications And Associated Conditions

Potential Complications Of Inflammatory Bowel Disease

The consequences of Inflammatory Bowel Disease (IBD) are well-known and may affect organs other than the intestines. Even though gastrointestinal symptoms including diarrhea, abdominal discomfort, and rectal bleeding are often the main emphasis, IBD may present in a variety of other ways and impact multiple body areas. The quality of life of a patient may be greatly impacted by these consequences, which need thorough care.

The formation of fistulas and strictures within the gastrointestinal system is one of the most frequent side effects. Bowel blockages may result from constricted sections of the intestines, often caused by long-term inflammation and scarring.

Contrarily, fistulas are improper connections between the intestines and other organs or between various portions of the intestines, which cause the contents of the intestines to seep into the surrounding tissues. Surgery may be required as a result of these consequences to relieve symptoms and stop other issues.

Moreover, malabsorption, insufficient intake, or elevated nutrient needs from chronic inflammation put people with IBD at risk for nutritional deficiencies. Deficiencies in vital vitamins and minerals, such as calcium, iron, vitamin B12, and vitamin D, may cause a variety of symptoms, from weakness and exhaustion to bone diseases like osteoporosis.

IBD-related inflammation may also impact the liver, joints, eyes, and skin, leading to a variety of extraintestinal symptoms. Arthritis may induce joint discomfort and swelling, while skin disorders such as erythema nodosum and pyoderma gangrenosum can manifest as painful nodules or ulcers. Uveitis and scleritis are examples of ocular symptoms that may cause pain in the eyes and visual impairment. Furthermore, people with IBD are more likely to have liver inflammation, sometimes referred to as autoimmune hepatitis or primary sclerosing cholangitis (PSC), which calls for close observation and treatment.

The higher risk of colorectal cancer linked to chronic colon inflammation is another worrisome consequence. Individuals with ulcerative colitis in particular who have
a large colonic involvement need to have colonoscopies performed frequently for monitoring purposes. This is because early detection of cancer or precancerous alterations may lead to earlier management and better results.

All things considered, the possible consequences of IBD highlight how crucial it is to have complete treatment and ongoing monitoring to properly avoid and treat these negative effects. Individuals with IBD may lessen the negative effects of these issues on their health and well-being by using a multidisciplinary strategy that includes gastroenterologists, dietitians, surgeons, and other medical professionals.

Extraintestinal Manifestations

The effects of Inflammatory Bowel Disease (IBD) may extend outside the gastrointestinal tract and impact different organs and systems in the body, resulting in extraintestinal symptoms that often need specialist care. These manifestations may precede or occur simultaneously with gastrointestinal symptoms, and they may have a substantial influence on a patient's quality of life.

Arthritis is one of the most prevalent extraintestinal symptoms of inflammatory bowel disease (IBD). It may cause pain, swelling, and stiffness in big joints including the knees, ankles, and elbows. Peripheral arthritis is a kind of arthritis that is more common in people with Crohn's disease than ulcerative colitis and is often associated with intestinal disease activity. Apart from peripheral arthritis, axial arthritis may also affect the spine and sacroiliac joints in people with IBD, resulting in stiffness and discomfort in the lower back.

Another common occurrence in IBD patients is skin symptoms, which may range from minor rashes to more serious diseases. Painful, red nodules that usually occur on the shins and may be connected to an active illness are the hallmarks of erythema nodosum. Pyoderma gangrenosum often affects the lower limbs and manifests as painful ulcers with weak boundaries.

The quality of life of a patient may be greatly affected by these skin manifestations, which may need a dermatologist's advice for appropriate care.

IBD patients may also develop uveitis, episcleritis, and scleritis, among other ocular consequences, in addition to arthritis and skin symptoms. Inflammation of the middle layer of the eye, or uveitis, may result in discomfort, redness, and impaired vision. To avoid long-term consequences, uveitis requires immediate ophthalmologic assessment and treatment. Both scleritis and episcleritis, which are inflammations of the outer layers of the eye, may have similar symptoms and need specific treatment to reduce pain and maintain vision.

Additionally, autoimmune hepatitis and primary sclerosing cholangitis (PSC) are two liver-related problems that may result from IBD's impact on the hepatobiliary system. The hallmark of autoimmune hepatitis is immune-mediated inflammation of the liver, which, if unchecked, may lead to cirrhosis and liver failure. PSC causes the bile ducts to become inflamed and scarred, which eventually causes bile duct strictures and liver damage. It is important to closely monitor liver function tests and imaging investigations to diagnose and treat these problems as soon as possible.

All things considered, the extraintestinal symptoms of IBD highlight the systemic character of the illness and the need for a multidisciplinary approach to treatment. Healthcare professionals may enhance the quality of life and maximize outcomes for patients with inflammatory bowel disease (IBD) by attending to both gastrointestinal symptoms and extraintestinal signs.

Screening For Associated Conditions

There is a link between Inflammatory Bowel Disease (IBD) and a higher chance of acquiring extra-gastrointestinal health issues. For early identification and prompt intervention, screening for these related disorders is crucial, which will enhance the quality of life and results for people with IBD. When screening patients with IBD for related illnesses, medical professionals usually use a mix of clinical assessment, blood testing, imaging investigations, and endoscopic examination.

Osteoporosis, which is characterized by reduced bone density and an increased risk of fracture, is one of the most prevalent related disorders in people with IBD. In this group, osteoporosis develops as a result of corticosteroid usage, chronic inflammation, malabsorption of calcium and vitamin D, and immobility. To evaluate bone density and fracture risk, dual-energy X-ray absorptiometry

(DXA) testing is often used in osteoporosis screening. For those with IBD, pharmaceutical therapies, calcium and vitamin D supplements, and lifestyle changes may be advised to prevent or treat osteoporosis.

Colorectal cancer is another significant comorbidity, especially in those with long-term ulcerative colitis affecting the colon. In this demographic, the risk of colorectal cancer is higher due to chronic inflammation and dysplasia, a precancerous condition. If a person has a high risk of colon cancer or has many biopsies, regular surveillance colonoscopies are advised to identify dysplastic alterations or early-stage cancer. Timely intervention, including surgical resection or endoscopic mucosal resection, may enhance prognosis and improve outcomes when detected early.

In addition, autoimmune diseases including psoriasis, rheumatoid arthritis, and autoimmune thyroid disease are more common in people with IBD. Assessing clinical symptoms, doing lab tests, and sending patients to specialized care providers for further assessment and treatment are some of the steps in the screening process for these illnesses. For those with inflammatory bowel disease (IBD), prompt identification and treatment of related autoimmune illnesses may help reduce symptoms and enhance general health outcomes.

In addition, since IBD is a chronic illness, its effects on day-to-day functioning, and its stigma, mental health issues such as depression, anxiety, and adjustment disorders are common in people with IBD. Healthcare professionals may identify people at risk and provide the right support and solutions by conducting routine mental health screenings, either with structured interviews or self-report questionnaires. Patients with IBD may benefit from collaborative treatment that includes mental health specialists like psychologists or psychiatrists to address these problems and enhance their general well-being.

In general, complete treatment and management of patients with IBD need screening for related illnesses. Early diagnosis and treatment of these diseases allow medical professionals to reduce risks, improve treatment plans, and enhance the quality of life for IBD patients.

Preventive Measures

The chronic illness known as inflammatory bowel disease (IBD) is defined by inflammation of the gastrointestinal system, which often results in several problems and related illnesses. Prevention is key to lowering complications and enhancing overall health outcomes for IBD patients, even while therapeutic approaches concentrate on decreasing inflammation and symptomatology. These preventative strategies include vaccinations, medication management, lifestyle changes, and routine monitoring.

For those with IBD, dietary changes may aid with inflammation reduction and symptom relief. There isn't a single diet that works for everyone with IBD, although some individuals may find relief from symptoms like bloating, diarrhea, and stomach discomfort by following a certain carbohydrate or low-FODMAP diet. To avoid nutritional deficiencies and promote general health, it's also critical to make sure you're getting enough vitamins and minerals. Individuals with IBD may create customized food regimens that fit their unique requirements and preferences by speaking with a qualified dietitian or nutritionist.

Furthermore, as smoking has been connected to an increased risk of complications, increased drug needs, and illness flares, quitting smoking is crucial for anybody with IBD, especially those with Crohn's disease. By putting smoking cessation programs into place and offering tools for support, people may stop smoking and see improvements in their general health.

Another important preventative strategy for people with IBD is vaccination, as immunosuppressive drugs or weakened immune systems might put them at higher risk of infection. For people with IBD, routine immunizations against influenza, pneumococcal disease, and hepatitis B are advised to lower their risk of vaccine-preventable illnesses and their related consequences. Healthcare professionals should advise patients on the timing and safety of vaccines as well as make sure they are up to date on their immunizations.

For those with IBD, medication management is crucial to avoiding problems and illness flare-ups. Immunomodulators and biologic medicines are examples of maintenance drugs that help keep the illness in remission and manage inflammation, therefore lowering the risk of complications and hospital stays. The key to maximizing treatment results and stopping the development of illness is adherence to recommended prescription regimens and regular follow-up visits with healthcare professionals.

For those with IBD, routine surveillance and monitoring are essential parts of preventative management. Careful observation of disease activity, inflammatory indicators, nutritional condition, and adverse drug reactions enables medical professionals to make necessary treatment plan adjustments and to intervene early. Routine screening also improves overall health outcomes for

IBD patients by enabling early identification and prompt care for related illnesses including osteoporosis, colorectal cancer, and mental health issues.

In conclusion, taking preventative actions is essential for lowering the likelihood of complications and enhancing general health outcomes for those who have inflammatory bowel disease. Through the implementation of lifestyle adjustments, vaccine compliance assurance, medication management optimization, and routine monitoring and surveillance, healthcare practitioners may enable patients to take charge of their health and lead more fulfilling lives.

CHAPTER 8

Pregnancy And Family Planning

Fertility Considerations

For those who have inflammatory bowel disease (IBD), fertility may be a major issue, but it's important to realize that having IBD doesn't always equate to infertility. There are a few things to bear in mind, however.

First and foremost, it's important to discuss your want to get pregnant with your healthcare professional. They may give advice unique to your circumstances. To maximize your chances of conception while treating your IBD efficiently, they could suggest particular drugs or changes to your treatment plan.

IBD patients' infertility may sometimes be caused by the illness itself or by prior surgical procedures. For instance, scarring from surgery or pelvic inflammation may affect a woman's ability to conceive. Seeking advice from a fertility professional might help you investigate alternatives like assisted reproductive technology if you have worries about your ability to conceive.

Reproductive health also depends on maintaining general health. This includes maintaining a healthy diet, controlling stress, exercising often, and abstaining from behaviors like smoking that may hurt fertility.

Pregnancy And Disease Management

IBD sufferers may have particular difficulties during pregnancy, although most women may have healthy pregnancies with proper preparation and treatment. Collaboration with your healthcare team is crucial throughout your pregnancy.

It's critical to have well-controlled IBD before pregnancy. This might include changing prescriptions or treatment regimens to reduce the possibility of flare-ups during pregnancy. Throughout pregnancy, it is crucial to regularly evaluate disease activity and symptoms to swiftly manage any concerns that may arise.

Some women may notice changes in their IBD symptoms during pregnancy. Some people could see an improvement, while others might have flare-ups. To guarantee timely management and necessary treatment modifications, it is imperative that you express any changes or concerns to your healthcare professional.

In some situations, it may be necessary to modify medicine during pregnancy to protect the mother and unborn child. However many of the drugs used to treat IBD are safe to use while pregnant, and the dangers of leaving the illness untreated often exceed the risks of taking the drugs.

Medication Safety During Pregnancy And Breastfeeding

A large number of people with IBD depend on drugs to control their symptoms and keep them in remission. Nonetheless, questions about these drugs' safety during pregnancy and nursing are often raised.

It is important that you and your healthcare practitioner talk about drug safety before becoming pregnant. They may provide advice on which drugs are safe to use while pregnant and which ones might need to be changed or stopped.

Certain biologics and immunomodulators, which are often used to treat IBD, are generally regarded as safe to use when pregnant or nursing. Some, nonetheless, could pose dangers.

Whether to continue taking a drug or stop taking it altogether should be decided case-by-case after considering the advantages and disadvantages for the mother and the unborn child.

Many IBD drugs may, in trace levels, enter breast milk while nursing. Even though the majority are thought to be safe, it's crucial to share any worries with your healthcare professional to guarantee the greatest treatment for you and your child.

Supportive Care For Expectant Mothers

Anyone may find pregnancy to be difficult, but those who have IBD may have extra worries and pressures. Prioritizing self-care and getting help when required is crucial throughout the pregnancy experience.

Counseling or therapy may be part of supportive treatment for pregnant moms with IBD to address any emotional or psychological difficulties associated with managing a chronic disease during pregnancy. Making connections with other IBD-afflicted women who have experienced pregnancy may also be a great source of support and direction.

Furthermore, sustaining a healthy lifestyle throughout pregnancy may enhance general well-being. This includes frequent exercise, getting enough sleep, and practicing stress management. It's important to pay attention to your body and be honest with your healthcare practitioner about any worries or difficulties you may be experiencing. Most IBD women can have successful pregnancies and healthy infants with the right care and assistance.

CHAPTER 9

Research And Innovations

Advancements In Inflammatory Bowel Disease Research

Recent years have witnessed impressive developments in the field of research on Inflammatory Bowel Disease (IBD), providing hope to millions of people afflicted with these chronic illnesses. Researchers and healthcare providers have been exploring the complex processes that underlie IBD to provide more potent therapies and enhance the quality of life for their patients.

Understanding the intricate interactions between genetics, the immune system, and environmental variables in the development of IBD is one important area of study. Numerous genetic variations have been linked to an elevated risk of IBD by researchers using genome-wide association studies (GWAS) and other genetic investigations. This information offers insights into possible therapy targets in addition to helping with early diagnosis and risk assessment.

Furthermore, discoveries in immunology and molecular biology have revealed important inflammatory pathways connected to the pathophysiology of IBD. Understanding the functions of different cytokines, signaling molecules, and immune cells has allowed researchers to create tailored medications that precisely alter these pathways, resulting in more specialized and efficient medical interventions.

Furthermore, our knowledge of the gut microbiome's function in IBD has completely changed with the development of high-throughput sequencing technology.

Research has shown dysbiosis, or imbalance, in the gut microbial community of IBD patients, pointing to a possible connection between the development of the illness and the makeup of the microbiota. As a result, new treatment approaches have surfaced that target the restoration of microbial equilibrium. These include probiotics, prebiotics, and fecal microbiota transplantation (FMT).

Apart from biological studies, advancements in diagnostic procedures and imaging modalities have made early illness identification and monitoring easier. Non-invasive methods of seeing the gastrointestinal system, such as capsule endoscopy and magnetic resonance enterography (MRE), can evaluate disease activity and consequences.

Overall, the subject of IBD has advanced due to the synergy of multidisciplinary research efforts, which have provided new understandings of disease processes and treatment opportunities.

The future of IBD research is bright, with studies into genetics, immunology, microbiology, and clinical outcomes still underway.

Promising Therapies And Treatment Approaches

To minimize side effects and address the underlying processes of inflammation, promising new therapeutic options for Inflammatory Bowel Disease (IBD) have emerged. The goal of these techniques is to establish long-term remission.

The development of biologic agents—engineered proteins that selectively target important components involved in the inflammatory cascade—is one noteworthy development in the treatment of inflammatory bowel disease (IBD). Because they provide strong and focused reduction of inflammation, biologics such as integrin antagonists, interleukin-12/23 inhibitors, and tumor necrosis factor-alpha (TNF-α) inhibitors have completely changed the way that IBD is managed. These drugs have shown promise in relieving symptoms, bringing patients into and keeping them in remission, and lowering the need for corticosteroids and hospital stays.

In addition, another type of medicine that shows promise for managing IBD is small molecule inhibitors. Small molecules are oral medications that block certain intracellular signaling pathways connected to inflammation, in contrast to biologics, which are big proteins given by injection or infusion. For example, cytokine signaling pathways are disrupted by Janus kinase (JAK) inhibitors, which reduce the inflammatory response. Patients with moderate to severe IBD have shown success with these oral medicines, which also provide convenience and flexibility in therapy administration.

Personalized medicine techniques are also becoming more popular in the treatment of IBD; they try to customize therapy according to the unique features of each patient, such as their genetic profile, disease phenotype, and response to treatment. Clinicians may maximize therapy effectiveness and minimize side effects by optimizing medication selection and dose via the integration of clinical data, biomarkers, and genetic information.

Furthermore, complementary therapy and lifestyle changes are essential to the comprehensive care of IBD. In some cases, dietary therapies like the low-FODMAPS diet or exclusive enteral nutrition (EEN) may help lower inflammation and relieve symptoms. Probiotics, acupuncture, yoga, and other complementary therapies may also be used in conjunction with traditional medical treatments to promote general well-being and manage symptoms.

To summarize, the growing array of medications and treatment modalities provides people with IBD with fresh hope. Future developments in clinical trials and research might lead to even more individualized, comprehensive, and successful approaches to enhance the quality of life and results for individuals suffering from chronic inflammatory disorders.

Clinical Trials And Patient Participation

Vital components of medical research, clinical trials provide a means of assessing the effectiveness and safety of new therapies and interventions for Inflammatory Bowel Disease (IBD). Patients who take part in clinical trials not only get access to state-of-the-art medications, but they also help to further medical research and provide better treatments for coming generations.

A broad spectrum of experimental treatments, such as immune modulators, biological medicines, small molecule inhibitors, and targeted therapy, are investigated in IBD clinical trials. These studies might assess how well novel drugs work to lower inflammation, induce and sustain remission, stop health problems, or enhance patients' quality of life.

Clinical trial participation is voluntary and subject to informed consent, which is obtained when participants are fully told about the study's goals, methods, possible risks and benefits, and their legal rights as research subjects. Patients are screened before participation to make sure they satisfy certain eligibility requirements based on things like the severity of the condition, prior treatment history, and general health.

To evaluate therapy response, keep an eye out for unfavorable occurrences, and guarantee patient safety, participants in the experiment are closely supervised and monitored by medical professionals. Participants may be subjected to a variety of evaluations, such as physical exams, laboratory testing, imaging investigations, and patient-reported outcome measures, depending on the research design.

Furthermore, it is becoming more widely acknowledged that patient involvement and feedback are essential to the planning and conduct of clinical trials. To ensure that clinical trials meet patients' most urgent needs and concerns, patient advisory boards, advocacy organizations, and patient-centered research efforts are essential in determining research priorities.

Patients who actively participate in clinical trials not only have access to potentially life-changing medications, but they also add to the body of information that will shape future developments in the treatment of IBD. In the end, innovation and advancement in the hunt for improved therapies and eventually an IBD cure are fueled by patient, researcher, and healthcare provider cooperation.

Future Directions In Disease Management

Prospects for improving patient care, enhancing treatment approaches, and comprehending the underlying processes of Inflammatory Bowel Disease (IBD) are bright. In IBD research and clinical practice, new trends and directions are being pursued to address existing issues and enhance the lives of those who suffer from these inflammatory chronic illnesses.

Personalized medicine is a major area of attention, whereby treatment choices are made based on specific patient features, such as illness phenotype, genetic makeup, and therapeutic response. Clinicians can maximize therapy effectiveness while reducing side effects by optimizing medication selection and dose via the integration of clinical data with biomarkers and genetic information.

Moreover, the development of precision medicine techniques seeks to pinpoint and uncover certain biological pathways linked to the pathophysiology of IBD. Researchers are using genomic profiling to uncover new therapeutic targets for intervention and to investigate the genetic basis of IBD. Targeted and customized treatments for inflammatory bowel disease (IBD) may be possible using precision medicines, which include gene editing tools like CRISPR-Cas9. These therapies can precisely modify genes and pathways linked to the illness.

Furthermore, there is increasing interest in using the gut microbiome's medicinal potential to address

IBD. Microbiota-based therapeutics and microbial metabolite modulation are two strategies that attempt to restore microbial balance and provide new ways to control inflammation and support mucosal repair in the gastrointestinal system.

Furthermore, improvements in digital health technology might improve IBD patient engagement, illness monitoring, and remote treatment delivery. Through the use of wearable technology, telemedicine platforms, and mobile health apps, patients may take an active role in their care and increase treatment adherence by making use of real-time symptom monitoring, remote consultations, and tailored health coaching.

CHAPTER 10

Advocacy And Awareness

Advocacy Initiatives For Inflammatory Bowel Disease

To guarantee that individuals with inflammatory bowel disease (IBD) get the assistance, resources, and care they need, advocacy is essential. Organizations, patient groups, and private citizens all take different steps to promote improved knowledge, care, and assistance for patients with IBD.

Pushing for more financing for IBD research and medical services is a big part of advocacy. To give IBD top priority on the healthcare agenda entails interacting with legislators at the local, national, and worldwide levels. Advocates often try to educate lawmakers about the difficulties IBD patients encounter and the value of funding support services and research.

To make sure that IBD patients' demands are sufficiently met by the healthcare system, advocacy also includes working with medical personnel. This might include promoting better access to expert care, available treatment alternatives, and supporting services including dietary counseling and mental health counseling.

Furthermore, by increasing knowledge and promoting understanding in the larger society, advocacy initiatives seek to lessen the stigma associated with IBD. Advocates work to debunk myths and misunderstandings around IBD by using a variety of media outlets, sharing personal experiences, and planning educational events.

This helps to foster a stronger sense of acceptance and support for those who are living with the illness.

Raising Awareness In The Community

Educating the public about Inflammatory Bowel Disease (IBD) is crucial to building compassion, empathy, and community support. To reach a variety of audiences and provide accurate information about the illness, advocates use a variety of tactics.

Public education initiatives are one method of increasing awareness. These campaigns disseminate information on IBD, including its symptoms, diagnosis, and available treatments, using traditional and digital media channels. Advocates may also plan neighborhood activities like walks, fundraisers, and educational sessions to interact with the public directly and provide forums for discussion and education.

Social media advocates may reach a wide range of audiences and share educational materials and personal stories, which is crucial in increasing public awareness about IBD. Through hashtags, online communities, and specialized advocacy sites, people with IBD may interact with one another, exchange information, and make their voices heard by a larger audience.

Healthcare facilities, businesses, and educational institutions are all excellent ways to spread knowledge about IBD. To increase awareness and empathy among students, coworkers, and healthcare professionals, advocates may engage with educators, employers, and healthcare providers to include IBD education in the curriculum, workplace wellness initiatives, and patient support services.

Supporting Research And Education Efforts

Promoting research and educational programs is essential to improving our knowledge of and ability to manage inflammatory bowel disease (IBD). Collaborating with academics, healthcare professionals, and organizations, advocates provide funding for research initiatives, provide teaching materials, and spread knowledge to the public and healthcare sectors.

Raising money for grants and scholarships that allow researchers to work with physicians and scientists to improve IBD diagnosis, treatment, and management is one method supporters promote research in this area. This money may also go toward projects that look into possible treatments, look into the fundamental causes of IBD, and improve patient outcomes.

Additionally, advocates are essential in informing medical practitioners about the most recent developments in IBD research and clinical practice. Advocates provide opportunities for cooperation and information sharing amongst gastroenterologists, nurses, dietitians, and other healthcare professionals engaged in IBD treatment by planning conferences, seminars, and continuing education courses.

Additionally, advocates create and disseminate educational resources to help patients and their families better understand IBD and give them the authority to make choices about their treatment. Brochures, films, internet courses, and support groups are a few examples of these tools that guide symptom management, choosing a treatment plan, and obtaining support services.

Empowering Patients To Be Advocates

A key component of advocacy work is enabling patients to speak out on behalf of other people with IBD and themselves. Advocates empower patients to take an active role in decision-making, get access to resources, and speak out for their needs in the healthcare system and the larger community by providing them with information, skills, and support.

A key element of patient empowerment is education. By educating patients about their conditions, available treatments, and self-management techniques, advocates enable patients to actively participate in their healthcare process. Individualized internet resources, instructional courses, and one-on-one therapy may be used to meet the unique requirements and preferences of each patient.

Apart from providing knowledge, advocates also help and motivate patients to deal with the difficulties of having IBD. Peer mentorship programs, support groups, and online communities are some of the ways that patients may find individuals who are similar to them and exchange helpful coping mechanisms for symptoms and treatment-related concerns.

Advocates also help individuals have the chance to tell their stories and speak out for themselves and other IBD sufferers. Through media appearances, public speaking engagements, or involvement in advocacy campaigns, sufferers possess a potent platform to generate consciousness, foster comprehension, and bring about constructive alterations in policies and procedures concerning IBD treatment and assistance.

CONCLUSION

In summary, IBD—also known as inflammatory bowel disease—poses a complex challenge to healthcare professionals, patients, and carers. It is clear from this investigation that managing IBD needs a multifaceted strategy that includes dietary, psychosocial, and medicinal assistance.

First and foremost, the goals of medical therapies, which include medication and surgical procedures, are to relieve symptoms, create and sustain remission, and avoid complications including strictures and fistulas. Biologics and immunomodulators are examples of medication treatments that have advanced and show promise in reducing inflammation and enhancing patient quality of life.

Second, diet is very important for the management of IBD. Although there isn't one diet that works for everyone with IBD, certain dietary adjustments, such as low-residue, low-FODMAP, or particular carbohydrate diets, may assist with symptoms and inflammation reduction. Furthermore, nutritional supplements could be required to treat vitamin deficits and malnutrition, which are often linked to IBD.

Moreover, the psychosocial consequences of IBD are indescribable. The disease's unpredictable course, severe symptoms, and chronic nature may cause anxiety, sadness, and a decline in social functioning. Therefore, it is crucial to include psychological support services, such as counseling and support groups, while managing the mental health of IBD patients.

To put it simply, managing IBD requires a comprehensive strategy that takes into account the interactions between dietary, psychological, and medical aspects. Through the implementation of a multidisciplinary approach that integrates nutritional therapies, medical treatment, and psychological support, healthcare professionals may maximize results and improve the general well-being of people with IBD. It is crucial to keep an eye out for new treatment modalities and holistic methods to enhance patient care and results as research into IBD progresses and our knowledge of the condition grows.

THE END